Seafood and Salads Cookbook for the Anti-Inflammatory Diet

Fantastic and Easy Fish Recipes That Will
Help You Reduce Inflammation
in Your Body

By
Olga Jones

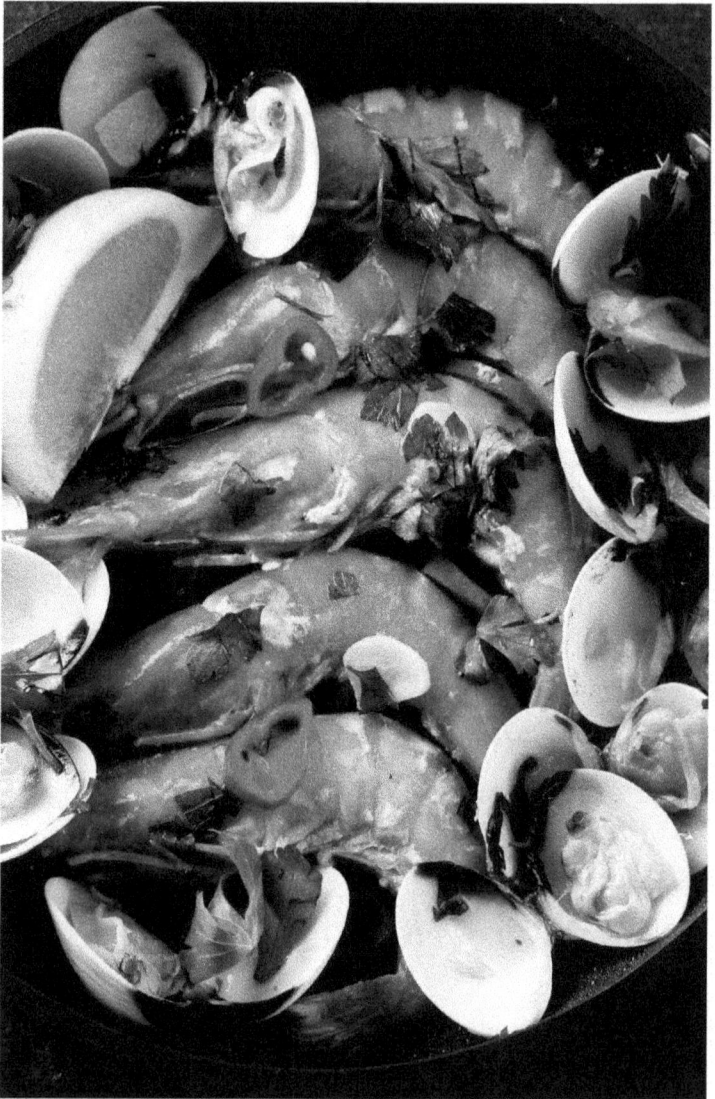

the publisher or the original author of this work can be in any fashion deemed liable for any hardship or damages that may befall them after undertaking information described herein.

Additionally, the information in the following pages is intended only for informational purposes and should thus be thought of as universal. As befitting its nature, it is presented without assurance regarding its prolonged validity or interim quality. Trademarks that are mentioned are done without written consent and can in no way be considered an endorsement from the trademark holder.

Table of Contents

INTRODUCTION

What is the Anti-Inflammatory Diet?

The anti-inflammatory diet is the best choice for your health if you have conditions that cause inflammation. Such conditions are asthma, chronic peptic ulcer, tuberculosis, rheumatoid arthritis, periodontitis, Crohn's disease, sinusitis, active hepatitis, etc. Along with medical treatment, proper nutrition is very important. An anti-inflammatory diet can help to reduce the pain from inflammation for a few notches. Such a diet isn't a panacea but a significant help in any treatment. Inflammation is a natural response of your body to infections, injuries, and illnesses. The classic symptoms of inflammation are redness, pain, heat, and swelling. Nevertheless, some diseases don't have any symptoms. Such illnesses are diabetes, heart disease, cancer, etc. That's why we should care about our health permanently and an anti-inflammatory diet is one of the ways for it.

Inflammation is your immune system's response to injury or unwanted microbes in your body. It is a natural process and vital part of your body's healing process. When inflammation becomes systemic and chronic, however, it becomes a problem, and measures need to be taken. This type of inflammation serves no purpose, and can cause a lot of harm to the body.

This book has a LOT of recipes, and not every recipe might work for you. For example, if you're allergic to dairy or gluten, the recipes containing those ingredients will cause more harm than good. However, substitutions are possible for all of these, so you will be fine following this book as long as you keep an eye on the ingredients and use a bit of creativity where you have to! Once you understand the fundamentals of the diet, you will be fully equipped to create your own recipes from scratch!This is the most important information that you should know before starting a diet. Any diet is not a magic remedy for all diseases; it is a support for the body during a difficult time of treatment. Start your new healthy life from one small step and you will see the huge results within half a year. You can be sure that your body will be thankful to you by giving you a fresh look and energy for new achievements.

Shrimp with Fruit & Bell Pepper

Yield: 4-6 servings
Preparation Time: 15 minutes
Cooking Time: 12 minutes

Ingredients:
- ½ cup onion, sliced thinly
- 1 teaspoon coconut oil
- 1½ pound shrimp, peeled and deveined
- ½ of red bell pepper, seeded and sliced thinly
- 1 mango, peeled, pitted and sliced
- 8-ounce can of pineapple tidbits with unswee10ed juice
- 1 cup coconut milk
- 1 tablespoon red curry paste
- 2 tablespoons fish sauce
- 2 tablespoons fresh cilantro, chopped

Directions:
1. Heat a nonstick pan on medium-high heat.
2. Add onion and sauté for approximately 3-4 minutes.
3. With a spoon, push the onion to the side of the pan.
4. Add coconut oil and shrimp and cook for about 2 minutes per side.
5. Add peppers and cook for approximately 3-4 minutes.

6. Add remaining ingredients except cilantro and simmer for approximately 5 minutes.

7. Serve hot using the sprinkling of cilantro.

Shrimp with Asparagus

Yield: 4 servings

Preparation Time: fifteen minutes

Cooking Time: 11 minutes

Ingredients:

- 2 tablespoons coconut oil
- 1 bunch asparagus, peeled and chopped
- 1 pound shrimp, peeled and deveined
- 4 garlic cloves, minced
- ½ teaspoon ground ginger
- 2 tablespoons fresh lemon juice
- 2/3 cup chicken broth

Directions:

1. In a big skillet, melt coconut oil on medium-high heat.

2. Add all ingredients except broth and cook for around 2 minutes, without stirring.

3. Stir and cook for around 5 minutes.

4. Add broth and cook for around 2-4 minutes.

5. Serve hot.

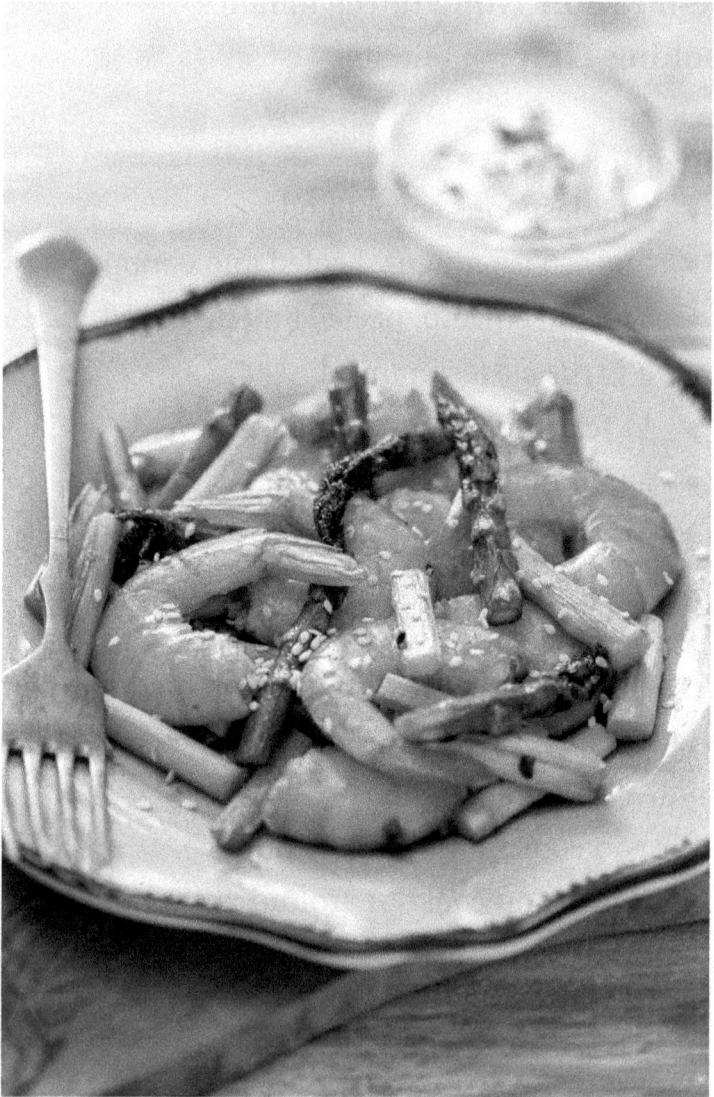

Pan Fried Squid

Yield: 2 servings

Preparation Time: quarter-hour

Cooking Time: 13 minutes

Ingredients:
- 1 teaspoon organic olive oil
- ¼ of yellow onion, sliced
- 1 pound squid, cleaned and cut into rings
- ¼ teaspoon ground turmeric
- Salt, to taste
- 1 organic egg, bea1o

Directions:
1. In a skillet, heat oil on medium-high heat.

2. Add onion and sauté for about 4-5 minutes.

3. Add squid rings, turmeric and salt and toss to coat well.

4. Reduce the temperature to medium-low and simmer for approximately 5 minutes.

5. Add bea1o eggs and cook, stirring continuously approximately 2-3 minutes.

6. Serve hot.

Scallops with Veggies

Yield: 1 serving

Preparation Time: 15 minutes

Cooking Time: 9 minutes

Ingredients:

- ½ cup unsalted vegetable broth, divided
- 1/3 cup carrot, peeled and chopped
- ¾ cup celery chopped
- 1 cup green beans, trimmed and chopped
- ¾ of green apple, cored and chopped
- ½ teaspoon fresh ginger herb, grated finely
- 1 teaspoon ground cardamom
- 1 teaspoon extra virgin olive oil
- 4-ounces sea scallops
- 1 tablespoon walnuts, chopped

Directions:

1. In a skillet, heat 3 tablespoons of broth and cook for approximately 4-5 minutes.

2. Stir in green beans, apple, ginger, cardamom and remaining broth and cook approximately 3-4 minutes.

3. Meanwhile in the frying pan, heat oil and cook the scallops for around 2-4 minutes per side.

4. Divide veggie mixture in serving plates.

5. Top with squid and serve.

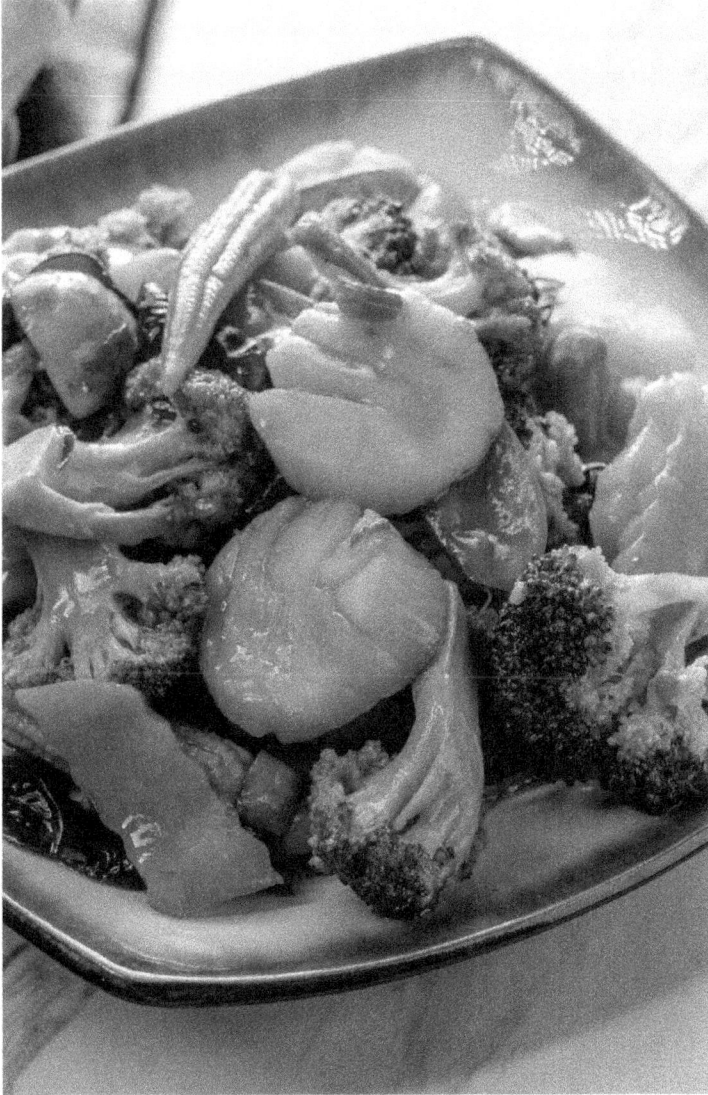

Spicy Scallops

Yield: 3-4 servings

Preparation Time: quarter-hour

Cooking Time: 13 minutes

Ingredients:

- 2 tablespoons coconut milk
- ½ cup shallot, minced
- ¼ cup tomato paste
- 2 teaspoons fresh ginger paste
- 2 teaspoons garlic paste
- ½ teaspoon garam masala
- ¼ teaspoon ground cinnamon
- ¼ teaspoon ground cumin
- Pinch of red pepper cayenne
- Salt, to taste
- 1 pound sea scallops
- 8-ounce plain Greek yogurt, whipped
- Chopped fresh cilantro, for garnishing

Directions:

1. In a large skillet, melt coconut oil on medium-high heat

2. Add shallots and sauté approximately 2-3 minutes.

3. Add remaining ingredients except scallops, yogurt and cilantro and cook for about 3-5 minutes.

4. Stir in scallops and yogurt and cook for approximately 5 minutes.

5. Serve hot using the garnishing of cilantro.

Spicy Kingfish

Yield: 2 servings
Preparation Time: fifteen minutes
Cooking Time: 10 min

Ingredients:

- 1 teaspoon dried unswee1oed coconut
- 1 teaspoon cumin seeds
- 1 teaspoon fennel seeds
- 1 teaspoon peppercorns
- 10 curry leaves
- ½ teaspoon ground turmeric
- 1½ teaspoons fresh ginger, grated finely
- 1 garlic herb, minced
- Salt, to taste
- 1 tablespoon fresh lime juice
- 4 (4-ounce) kingfish steaks
- 1 tbsp olive oil
- 1 lime wedge

Directions:

1. Heat a surefire skillet on low heat.

2. Add coconut, cumin seeds, fennel seeds, peppercorns and curry leaves and cook, stirring continuously for about 1 minute.

3. Remove in the heat and let it cool completely.

4. In a spice grinder, add the spice mixture and turmeric and grind rill powdered finely.

5. Transfer the mixture into a large bowl with ginger, garlic, salt and lime juice and mix well. 6. Add fish fillets and cat while using mixture evenly.

7. Refrigerate to marinate approximately 3 hours.

8. In a big nonstick skillet, heat oil on medium heat.

9. Add the fish fillets and cook for approximately 3-5 minutes per side or till desired doneness.

10. Transfer onto a paper towel lined plate to drain.

11. Serve with lime wedges.

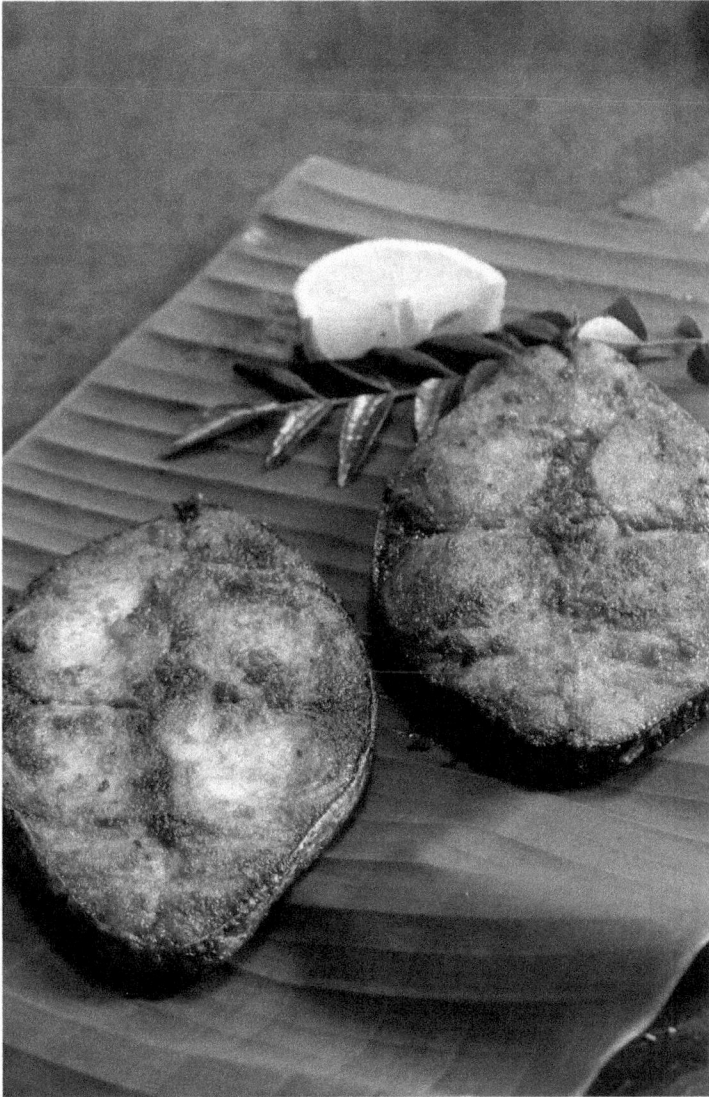

Spicy Salmon

Yield: 4 servings
Preparation Time: quarter-hour
Cooking Time: 7 minutes

Ingredients:

- Salt, to taste
- 2 small onions, chopped
- 2 large garlic cloves, chopped
- 1 (1- inch) piece fresh ginger, chopped
- 1 teaspoon ground turmeric
- 2 teaspoons red chili powder
- Salt and freshly ground black pepper, to taste
- 2 tablespoons fresh lemon juice
- 4 salmon steaks
- Coconut oil, as required for shallow frying

Directions:

1. In a food processor, add all ingredients except salmon and oil and pulse till smooth.

2. Transfer the mix right into a bowl.

3. Add steaks and coat with marinade generously.

4. Refrigerate to marinate for overnight.

5. In a large skillet, melt coconut oil on medium-high heat.

6. Add salmon fillet, skin-side up and cook for approximately 4 minutes.

7. Flip the medial side and cook for approximately 3 minutes.

8. Transfer onto a paper towel lined plate to drain.

9. Serve with lemon wedges.

Salmon with Cabbage

Yield: 4 servings

Preparation Time: fifteen minutes

Cooking Time: 10 minutes

Ingredients:

- 1 (1-inch) piece fresh ginger, grated finely
- 2 tablespoons raw honey
- 1 tablespoon freshly squeezed lemon juice
- 1 tablespoon Dijon mustard
- 4 tablespoons organic olive oil, divided
- 4 (8-ounce) salmon fillets
- 1 small head cabbage, sliced thinly
- 1 garlic clove, minced
- 1 tablespoon sesame seeds
- Freshly ground black pepper, to taste
- 4 scallions, chopped

Directions:

1. In a bowl, mix together ginger, honey, fresh lemon juice and Dijon mustard. Keep aside.

2. In a sizable nonstick skillet, heat 1 tablespoon of oil on medium high heat.

3. Add salmon and cook for around 3-4 minutes per side.

4. Place the honey mixture over salmon fillets evenly and immediately remove from heat.

5. Cover and make aside till serving.

6. Meanwhile in another skillet, heat 2 tablespoons of oil on medium heat.

7. Add cabbage and stir fry for approximately 3-4 minutes.

8. Add remaining oil and stir fry for around 5 minutes.

9. Add garlic, sesame seeds and black pepper and cook for about 1 minute.

10. Place salmon over cabbage and serve with garnishing of scallion.

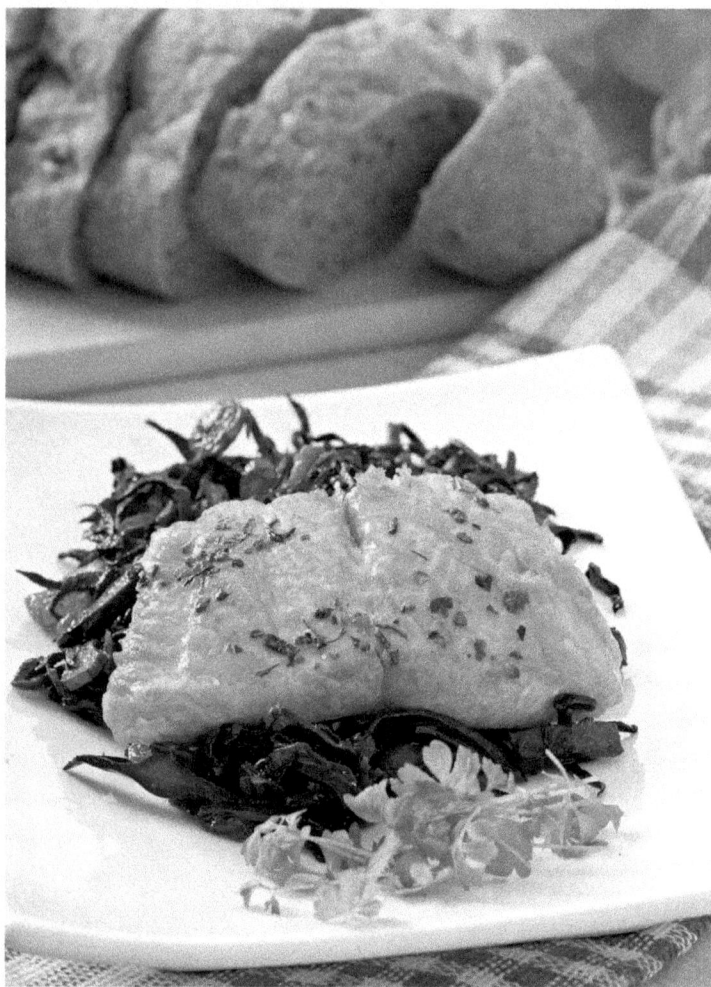

Basa with Mushroom & Bell Pepper

Yield: 2 servings

Preparation Time: quarter-hour

Cooking Time: 18 minutes

Ingredients:

- 1 (8-ounce) basa fish fillet, cubed
- ¼ teaspoon ginger paste
- ¼ teaspoon garlic paste
- 1 teaspoon red chili powder
- Salt, to taste
- 1 tablespoon coconut vinegar
- 1 tablespoon extra-virgin organic olive oil, divided
- ½ cup fresh mushrooms, sliced
- 1 small onion, quartered
- ¼ cup red bell pepper, seeded and cubed
- ¼ cup yellow bell pepper, seeded and cubed
- 2-3 scallions, chopped
- 1 teaspoon fish sauce

Directions:

1. In a bowl, mix together fish, ginger, garlic, chili powder and salt whilst aside for around twenty minutes.
2. In a nonstick skillet, heat 1 teaspoon of oil on medium-high heat.
3. Sear the fish for about 5-6 minutes or till golden coming from all sides.

4. In another skillet, heat remaining oil on medium heat.

5. Add mushrooms and onion and stir fry for about 5-7 minutes.

6. Add bell pepper and fish and stir fry for about 2 minutes.

7. Add scallion and fish sauce and stir fry for about 1-2 minutes.

8. Serve hot.

Snapper with Carrot & Broccoli

Yield: 2 servings

Preparation Time: quarter-hour

Cooking Time: 6 minutes

Ingredients:

- 2½ tbsp essential olive oil, divided
- 1 teaspoon red curry paste
- Salt, to taste
- 2 skinless snapper fillets
- 2 teaspoons coconut oil, divided
- ½ tablespoon fresh ginger, sliced thinly
- 10 baby carrots, peeled and halved
- 1 tablespoon fish sauce
- 1½ tablespoons freshly squeezed lemon juice, divided
- 1 teaspoon organic honey
- 2 cups broccoli florets
- Freshly ground black pepper, to taste
- 1 garlic cloves, minced

Directions:

1. In a bowl, mix together 2 tablespoons of essential olive oil, curry paste and salt.

2. Add snapper fillets and rub with oil mixture evenly. Keep aside for about 5-10 min.

3. In a small skillet, melt 1 teaspoon of coconut oil on medium heat.

4. Add ginger and carrots and stir fry for around 2 minutes.

5. Add fish sauce, 1 tablespoon of fresh lemon juice, honey and black pepper and stir fry approximately 2-3 minutes.

6. Meanwhile in another skillet, heat remaining olive oil on medium heat.

7. Add snapper fillets and cook for about 3 minutes from both sides.

8. Drizzle with remaining lemon juice.

9. Meanwhile in a pan of boiling water add broccoli and cook for around 2 minutes.

10. Drain well.

11. In a similar pan, melt remaining coconut oil on medium heat.

12. Add garlic and sauté for around 1 minute.

13. Add broccoli and toss to coat well.

14. Serve snapper fillets with carrots and broccoli.

Steamed Snapper Parcel

Yield: 2 servings

Preparation Time: fifteen minutes

Cooking Time: 10 min

Ingredients:

- 2 tablespoons garlic, minced
- 1 tablespoon fresh turmeric, grated finely
- 1 tablespoon fresh ginger, grated finely
- 2 tablespoons fresh lime juice
- 2 tablespoons coconut aminos
- 2 tablespoons essential olive oil
- 1 bunch fresh cilantro, chopped
- 2 (6-ounce) snapper fillets

Directions:

1. In a food processor, add garlic, turmeric, ginger, lime juice, coconut aminos and extra virgin olive oil and pulse till smooth.

2. Transfer a combination in the bowl with cilantro and mix well.

3. Add snapper fillets and coat using the mixture generously.

4. Place each fish fillet in the foil paper and wrap the paper to create a parcel.

5. Arrange a steamer basket inside a pan of boiling water.

6. Place the parcels in a steamer basket.

7. Cover and steam for about 10 min.

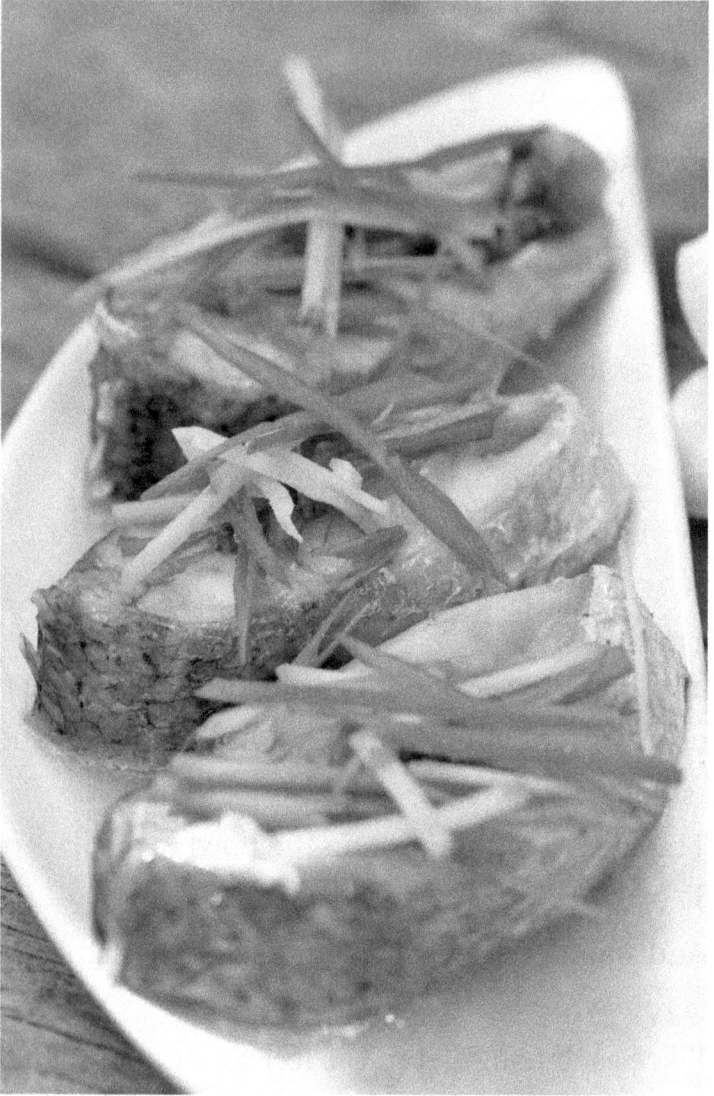

Broiled Sweet & Tangy Salmon

Yield: 3 servings

Preparation Time: quarter-hour

Cooking Time: 12 minutes

Ingredients:

- 2 garlic cloves, crushed
- 2 tablespoons fresh ginger grated finely
- 2 tablespoons organic honey
- 2 tablespoons coconut aminos
- 2 tablespoons fresh lime juice
- 3 tablespoons olive oil
- 3 tablespoons sesame oil
- 2 tablespoons black sesame seeds
- 1 tablespoon white sesame seeds
- 1 pound boneless salmon fillets
- 1/3 cup scallion, chopped

Directions:

1. In a baking dish, mix together all ingredients except the salmon. And scallion.
2. Add salmon and coat with mixture generously.
3. Refrigerate to marinate for about 40-45 minutes.
4. Preheat the broiler or oven and arrange the rack inside top in the oven.

5. Place the baking dish inside the oven and broil for approximately 10-12 minutes.

6. On a serving platter, put the salmon and top with all the pan sauce.

7. Serve while using garnishing of scallion.

Baked parsley Salmon

Yield: 3-4 servings

Preparation Time: fifteen minutes

Cooking Time: twenty or so minutes

Ingredients:

- 16-24-ounce salmon fillets
- 2 tablespoons coconut oil, melted
- 3 tablespoons fresh parsley, minced
- ¼ teaspoon ginger powder
- Salt, to taste

Directions:

1. Preheat the oven to 400 degrees F. Grease a substantial baking dish.

2. Arrange the salmon fillets into a prepared baking dish in a single layer.

3. Drizzle with coconut oil and sprinkle with parsley, ginger powder and salt.

4. Bake for about 15-twenty or so minutes.

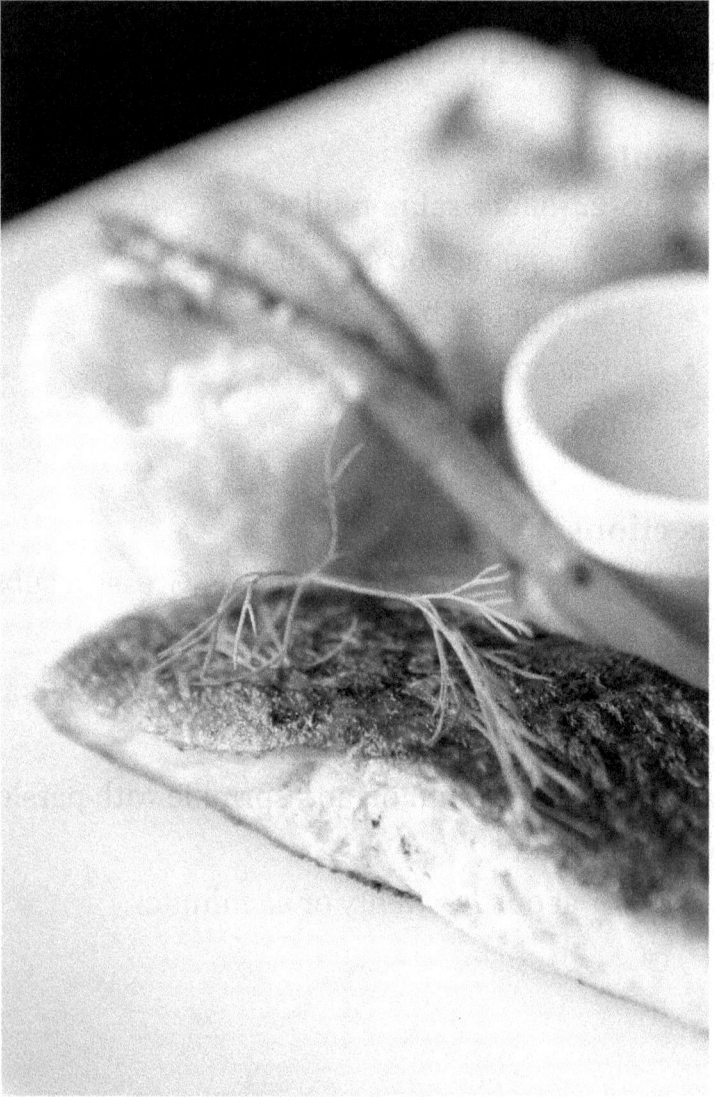

Baked Crispy Cod

Yield: 2-4 servings

Preparation Time: quarter-hour

Cooking Time: fifteen minutes

Ingredients:

- 1 green bell pepper, seeded and sliced
- 2 large eggs
- 1/3 cup blanched almond flour
- ¼ teaspoon dried dill weed, crushed
- ½ teaspoon garlic powder
- 1/8 teaspoon ground turmeric
- Freshly ground black pepper, to taste
- 1½ pound cod fillets
- Chopped fresh chives, for garnishing

Directions:

1. Preheat the oven to 350 degrees F. Line a large rimmed baking dish with parchment paper.

2. Arrange the bell pepper slices into the prepared baking dish.

3. In a shallow dish, crack the eggs and brat well.

4. In another shallow dish, mix together almond flour, dill weed, garlic powder, turmeric and black pepper.

5. Coat the cod fillets in egg and then roll into flour mixture evenly.

6. Place the cod fillets over bell pepper slices.

7. Bake for approximately fifteen minutes.

8. Serve with all the garnishing of chives.

Grilled Sweet & Tangy Salmon

Yield: 4 servings

Preparation Time: 15 minutes

Cooking Time: 15 minutes

Ingredients:

- 1 scallion, chopped
- 1 teaspoon garlic powder
- 1 teaspoon ground ginger
- ¼ cup organic honey
- 1/3 cup fresh orange juice
- 1/3 cup coconut aminos
- 1½ pound salmon fillets

Directions:

1. In a zip lock bag, add all ingredients and seal the bag.

2. Shake the bag to coat the mix with salmon.

3. Refrigerate for around thirty minutes, flipping occasionally.

4. Preheat the grill to medium heat. Grease the grill grate.

5. Remove the salmon from your bag, reserving the marinade.

6. Grill for around 10 minutes.

7. Coat the fillets with reserved marinade and grill for 5 minutes more.

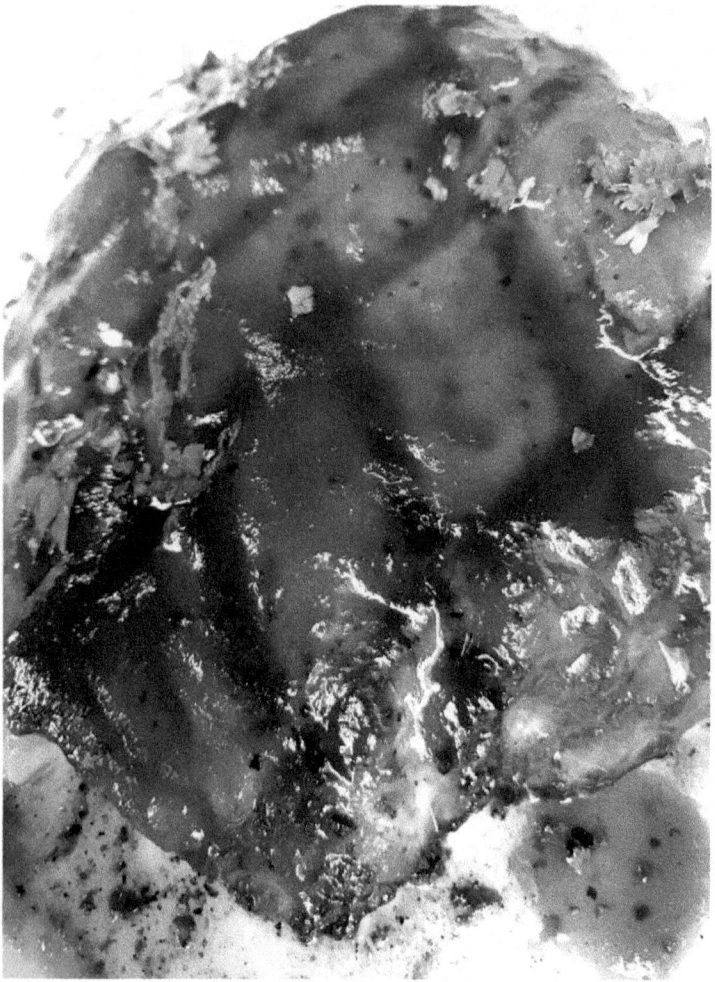

Grilled Spicy Salmon

Yield: 6-8 servings

Preparation Time: fifteen minutes

Cooking Time: 6-10 min

Ingredients:
- ½ tablespoon ground ginger
- ½ tablespoon ground coriander
- ½ tablespoon ground cumin
- ½ teaspoon paprika
- ¼ tsp red pepper cayenne
- Salt, to taste
- 1 tablespoon fresh orange juice
- 1 tablespoon coconut oil, melted
- 1½-2 pound salmon fillets

Directions:

1. In a big bowl, add all ingredients except salmon and mix till a paste forms.

2. Add salmon and coat with mixture generously.

3. Refrigerate to marinate for approximately thirty minutes.

4. Preheat the propane gas grill to high heat using the lid closed not less than 10 minutes.

5. Grease the grill grate, make the salmon fillets, skin-side down.

6. Cover with all the lid and grill for approximately 3 minutes.

7. Flip the medial side and cover while using the lid and grill for around 3 minutes more.

Rockfish Curry

Yield: 8 servings
Preparation Time: 15 minutes
Cooking Time: a half-hour

Ingredients:
- 2 pound rockfish
- ¾ teaspoon ground turmeric, divided
- Salt, to taste • 2 tablespoons coconut oil
- 12 pearl onions, halved
- 2 medium red onions, sliced thinly
- 2 Serrano peppers, halved
- 40 small leaves, divided
- 1 (½-inch) piece fresh ginger, minced
- Freshly ground black pepper, to taste
- ¼ cup water
- 1½ (14-ounce) cans coconut milk, divided
- 1 teaspoon using apple cider vinegar

Directions:
1. In a bowl, season the fish with ¼ teaspoon with the turmeric and salt whilst aside.
2. In a sizable skillet, melt coconut oil on medium heat.
3. Add pearl onions, red onions, ginger, Serrano peppers and 20 curry leaves and sauté approximately quarter-hour.
4. Add ginger, remaining turmeric, salt and black pepper and sauté for approximately 2 minutes.

5. Transfer half of the mixture into a bowl whilst aside.

6. Add remaining curry leaves, fish fillets, water and 1 can of coconut milk and cook for approximately 2 minutes.

7. Now cook, covered for approximately 5 minutes.

8. Add apple cider vinegar and remaining half can of coconut milk and cook for around 3-5 minutes or till done completely.

9. Serve hot using the topping of reserved onion mixture.

Lemony Shrimp

Yield: 4-6 servings
Preparation Time: quarter-hour
Cooking Time: 6 minutes

Ingredients:
- 1 small onion, chopped finely
- 1 tablespoon fresh ginger, minced
- 3 garlic cloves, minced
- 1 tablespoon fresh lemon zest, grated finely
- 1 fresh red chili, seeded and minced
- 1 teaspoon ground turmeric
- ½ cup olive oil
- ½ cup freshly squeezed lemon juice
- 20-24 raw shrimp, peeled and deveined
- 1 tablespoon coconut oil

Directions:
1. In a large bowl, mix together all ingredients except shrimp and coconut oil.

2. Add shrimp and coat with marinade generously.

3. Cover and refrigerate to marinate for overnight.

4. In a big nonstick skillet, melt coconut oil on medium high heat.

5. Transfer shrimp into skillet, reserving marinade.

6. Stir fry for around 3-4 minutes.

7. Ass reserved marinade and provide to a boil, tossing occasionally.

Shrimp with Broccoli

Yield: 2-4 servings

Preparation Time: 15 minutes

Cooking Time: 12 minutes

Ingredients:

- 1-2 tablespoons coconut oil, divided
- 4 cups broccoli, chopped
- 2 pound large shrimp, peeled and deveined
- 2 minced garlic cloves
- 1 (1-inch) piece fresh ginger, minced
- Salt and freshly ground black pepper, to taste

Directions:

1. In a substantial skillet, melt 1 tablespoon of coconut oil on medium-high heat.

2. Add broccoli and sauté for about 1-2 minutes.

3. Cover and cook, stirring occasionally for about 3-4 minutes.

4. With a spoon, push the onion to the side from the pan.

5. Add remaining coconut oil and let it melt.

6. Add shrimp and cook, tossing for approximately 2-3 minutes.

7. Add remaining ingredients and sauté approximately 2-3 minutes.

8. Serve hot.

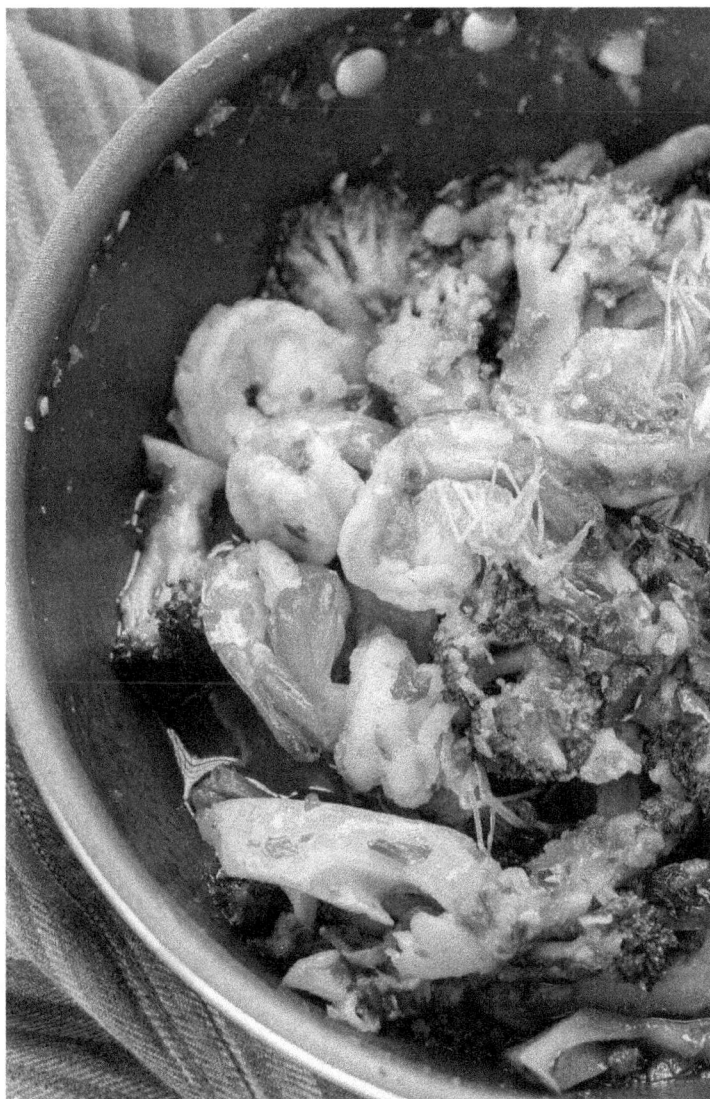

Prawns with Veggies

Yield: 4 servings
Preparation Time: fifteen minutes
Cooking Time: 9 minutes

Ingredients:
- 2 teaspoons coconut oil
- 1½ medium onions, sliced
- 1 tablespoon fresh ginger, grated finely
- 2 medium green peppers, sliced
- 3 medium carrots, peeled and sliced
- 1½ pound pawns, peeled and deveined
- 3 garlic cloves, minced
- 2½ teaspoons curry powder
- 1½ tablespoons fish sauce
- 1 cup coconut milk
- Water, as required
- Salt, to taste
- 2 tablespoons fresh lime juice

Directions:
1. In a large skillet, melt coconut oil on medium-high heat.
2. Add onion and sauté approximately 1 minute.
3. Add ginger, bell pepper and carrots and stir fry for about 2-3 minutes.

4. Add prawns, garlic, curry powder and fish sauce and stir fry for approximately a few seconds.

5. Add coconut milk plus a little water and stir fry approximately 3-4 minutes.

Squid with Veggies

Yield: 2 servings

Preparation Time: 20 minutes

Cooking Time: 10 min

Ingredients:

- 1 teaspoon extra virgin olive oil
- 2 carrots, peeled and chopped
- 2 red bell peppers, seeded and cut into strips
- ½ of eggplant, chopped
- ¾ pound squids, cleaned
- 2 tablespoons fish sauce
- 1 teaspoon fresh ginger, minced
- ½ teaspoon paprika
- 1 cup fresh spinach, chopped
- Salt and freshly ground black pepper, to taste
- 3 small zucchinis, spiralized with Blade C

Directions:

1. In a sizable skillet, heat oil on medium heat.

2. Add carrots, bell pepper and eggplant and stir fry for around 3-4 minutes.

3. Add remaining ingredients except zucchini and cook for about 1-2 minutes.

4. Stir in spinach and cook for approximately 3-4 minutes.

5. Meanwhile in a pan of boiling water, add zucchini noodles and cook for about 1 minute.

6. Drain well.

7. Transfer the zucchini noodles into two serving bowls.

8. Top with squid mixture and gently stir to blend.

9. Serve immediately.

Scallops with Broccoli

Yield: 2 servings

Preparation Time: fifteen minutes

Cooking Time: 6 minutes

Ingredients:

- ¼ cup fresh ginger, grated
- 8 large sea scallops
- 1 package frozen broccoli, thawed
- 1 tablespoon coconut oil
- Freshly ground black pepper, to taste

Directions:

1. In a pan of water, add ginger on medium heat.

2. Place scallops in the metal steamer basket and arrange inside the pan of water.

3. Cover and steam for approximately 2-5 minutes.

4. Meanwhile in another pan of boiling water, arrange the steamer basket.

5. Add broccoli and boil, covered for approximately 5 minutes.

6. Drain well.

7. In a sizable frying pan, melt coconut oil on medium heat.

8. Add scallops and sear for approximately thirty seconds from each party.

9. Serve the scallops over bed of broccoli.

10. Drizzle a little ginger water and serve.

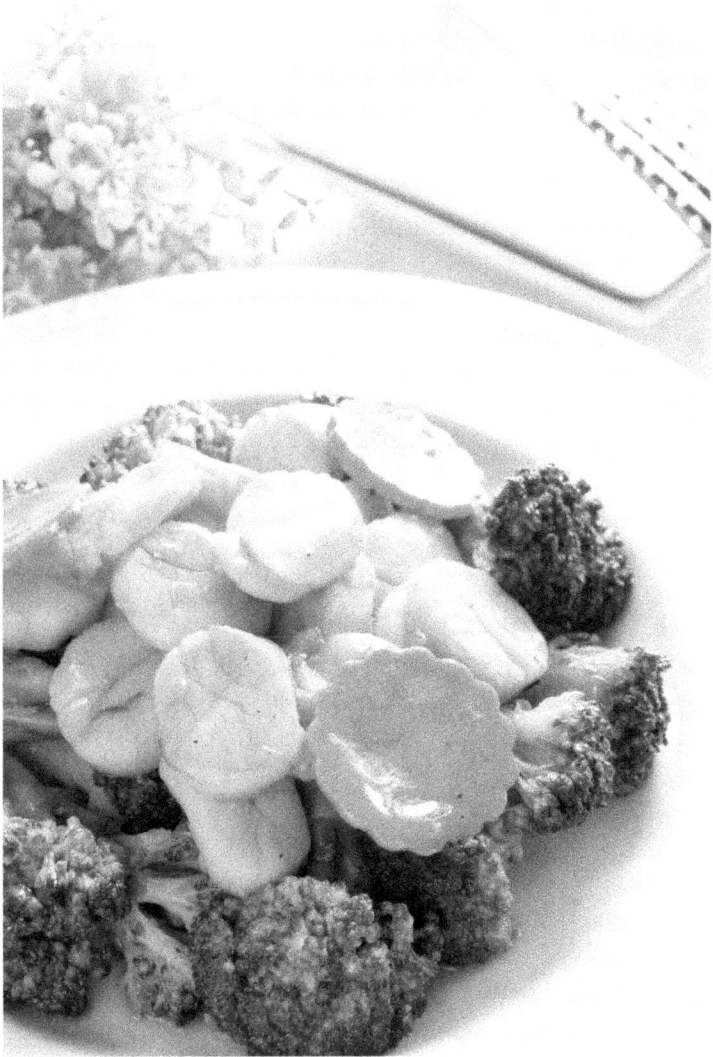

Deep Fried Kingfish

Yield: 4 servings

Preparation Time: fifteen minutes

Cooking Time: 8 minutes

Ingredients:

- ½ teaspoon ginger paste
- ½ teaspoon garlic paste
- 2 tablespoons chickpea flour
- 2 teaspoons turmeric powder
- 1 teaspoon ground coriander
- 1 teaspoon red chili powder
- ½ teaspoon garam masala
- Salt, to taste
- Water, as required
- 1 pound kingfisher fillets
- Olive oil, as necessary for deep frying

Directions:

1. In a large bowl, add all of the ingredients except the fish and oil and mix till a paste forms. 2. Add the fish fillets and coat using the paste generously.

3. Refrigerate to marinate for approximately 1 hour.

4. In a substantial deep skillet, heat oil on medium-high heat.

---

5. Add fish fillets and fry for about 3-4 minutes per side or till desired doneness.

6. Transfer onto a paper towel lined plate to drain.

Gingered Tilapia

Yield: 5 servings

Preparation Time: 15 minutes

Cooking Time: 6 minutes

Ingredients:
- 2 tablespoons coconut oil
- 5 tilapia fillets
- 3 garlic cloves, minced
- 2 tablespoons unsweetened coconut, shredded
- 4-ounce freshly ground ginger
- 2 tablespoons coconut aminos
- 8 scallions, chopped

Directions:
1. In a large skillet, melt coconut oil on medium heat.

2. Add tilapia fillets and cook for around 2 minutes.

3. Flip the inside and add garlic, coconut and ginger and cook for about 1 minute.

4. Add coconut aminos and cook for around 1 minute.

5. Add scallion and cook for approximately 1-2 minute more.

6. Serve immediately.

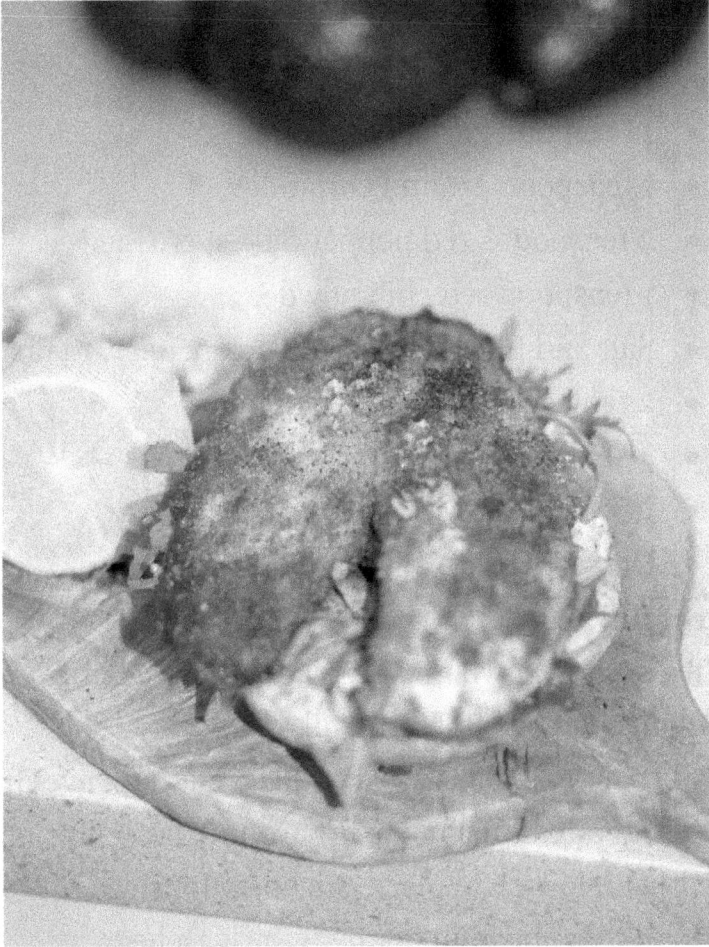

Crispy Salmon

Yield: 4 servings

Preparation Time: fifteen minutes

Cooking Time: 12 minutes

Ingredients:

- 1 teaspoon garlic powder
- 1 teaspoon ground coriander
- 2 teaspoons red pepper flakes, crushed
- 1 teaspoon red chili powder
- Salt and freshly ground black pepper, to taste
- 2 tablespoons fresh lemon juice
- 4 salmon steaks
- 1 cup chickpea flour
- Olive oil, as essential for deep frying

Directions:

1. In a sizable bowl, mix together all ingredients except salmon, chickpea flour and oil.

2. Add salmon steaks and coat with mixture evenly.

3. Refrigerate to marinate for around 3-4 hours.

4. In a shallow dish, place chickpea flour.

5. In a skillet, heat oil on medium-high heat.

6. Coat the salmon steaks with flour evenly.

7. Fry the salmon fillets approximately 5-6 minutes per side.

8. Transfer onto a paper towel lined plate to drain.

Salmon with Vegetables

Yield: 1 serving

Preparation Time: twenty minutes

Cooking Time: 19 minutes

Ingredients:

- 5 teaspoons extra virgin olive oil, divided
- 1 teaspoon ground turmeric
- 1 teaspoon paprika
- Salt and freshly ground black pepper, to taste
- 1 (4-ounce) salmon fillet
- 1 purple baby carrot, cut lengthwise
- 1 yellow carrot, cut lengthwise
- 1 orange carrot, cut lengthwise
- 3 French beans, chopped
- 3 button mushrooms, sliced

Directions:

1. In a bowl, mix together 2 teaspoons of oil, turmeric, paprika, salt and black pepper.

2. Add salmon and coat using the oil mixture evenly. Keep aside.

3. In a pan of boiling water, add French beans and carrots and cook for about 3 minutes.

4. Drain well.

5. In a nonstick skillet, heat 2 teaspoons of oil on medium heat.

6. Add mushroom and a pinch of salt and black pepper and stir fry for or about 5-6 minutes. 7. Add the drained vegetables and stir fry for approximately 2 minutes.

8. Transfer the vegetables onto a plate and loosely, cover having a foil paper to hold warm. 9. In a similar skillet, heat remaining oil on medium heat.

10. Add salmon fillet, skin-side down and cook for approximately 3-5 minutes.

11. Change the inside and cook for approximately 2-3 minutes.

12. Place salmon over vegetables and serve.

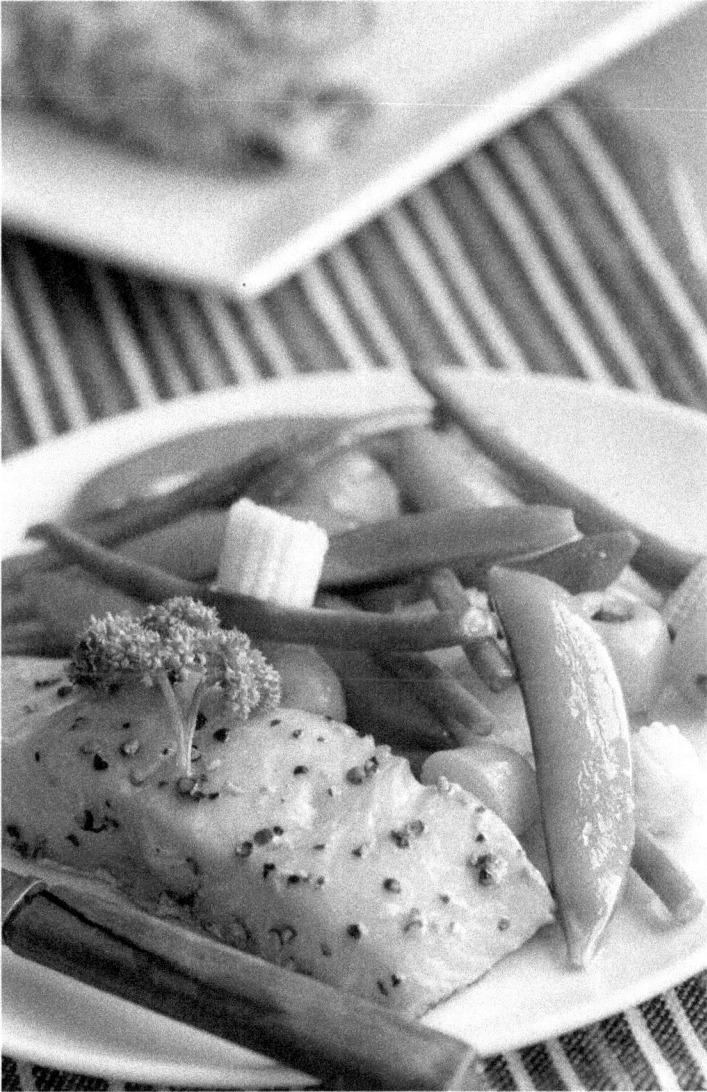

Haddock with Swiss Chard

Yield: 1 serving

Preparation Time: 15 minutes

Cooking Time: 10 minutes

Ingredients:
- 2 tablespoons coconut oil, divided
- 2 minced garlic cloves
- 2 teaspoons fresh ginger, grated finely
- 1 haddock fillet
- Salt and freshly ground black pepper, to taste
- 2 cups Swiss chard, chopped roughly
- 1 teaspoon coconut aminos

Directions:

1. In a skillet, melt 1 tablespoon of coconut oil on medium heat.

2. Add garlic and ginger and sauté approximately 1 minute.

3. Add haddock fillet and sprinkle with salt and black pepper.

4. Cook approximately 3-5 minutes per side or till desired doneness.

5. Meanwhile in another skillet, melt remaining coconut oil on medium heat.

6. Add Swiss chard and coconut aminos and cook for around 5-10 minutes.

7. Serve the salmon fillet over Swiss chard.

Citrus Poached Salmon

Yield: 3 servings
Preparation Time: fifteen minutes
Cooking Time: 12 minutes

Ingredients:
- 3 garlic cloves, crushed
- 1½ teaspoons fresh ginger, grated finely
- 1/3 cup fresh orange juice
- 3 tablespoons coconut aminos
- 3 (6-ounce) salmon fillets

Directions:
1. In a bowl, mix together all ingredients except salmon.

2. In the bottom of your large pan, squeeze salmon fillet.

3. Place the ginger mixture in the salmon and aside for about quarter-hour.

4. Place the pan on high heat and convey to your boil.

5. Reduce the heat to low and simmer, covered for about 10-12 minutes or till desired doneness.

Broiled Spicy Salmon

Yield: 4 servings

Preparation Time: fifteen minutes

Cooking Time: 14 minutes

Ingredients:

- ¼ cup low- Fat plain Greek yogurt
- ½ teaspoon ground coriander
- ½ teaspoon ground turmeric
- ½ teaspoon ground ginger
- ¼ tsp cayenne pepper
- Salt and freshly ground black pepper, to taste
- 4 (6-ounce) skinless salmon fillets

Directions:

1. Heat the broiler of the oven. Grease a broiler pan.

2. In a bowl, mix together all ingredients except the salmon.

3. Arrange salmon fillets onto the prepared broiler pan inside a single layer.

4. Place the yogurt mixture over each fillet evenly.

5. Broil approximately 12-14 minutes.

6. Serve immediately.

Baked Sweet Lemony Salmon

Yield: 2 servings
Preparation Time: 15 minutes
Cooking Time: 12 minutes

Ingredients:

- 2 (8-ounce) salmon fillets •
- ½ teaspoon organic honey and even more for drizzling
- 1/3 teaspoon ground turmeric, divided
- Freshly ground black pepper, to taste
- 2 large lemon slices

Directions:

1. In a zip lock bag, add salmon, ½ teaspoon of honey, ¼ teaspoon of turmeric and black pepper.

2. Seal the bag and shake to coat well.

3. Refrigerate to marinate for around 1 hour.

4. Preheat the oven to 40 degrees F.

5. Transfer the salmon fillets onto a cookie sheet in the single layer.

6. Cover the fillets with marinade.

7. Place the salmon fillets, skin-side up and bake for around 6 minutes.

8. Carefully, customize the side of fillets.

9. Sprinkle with remaining turmeric and black pepper evenly.

10. Place 1 lemon slice over each fillet and drizzle with honey.

11. Bake for approximately 6 minutes.

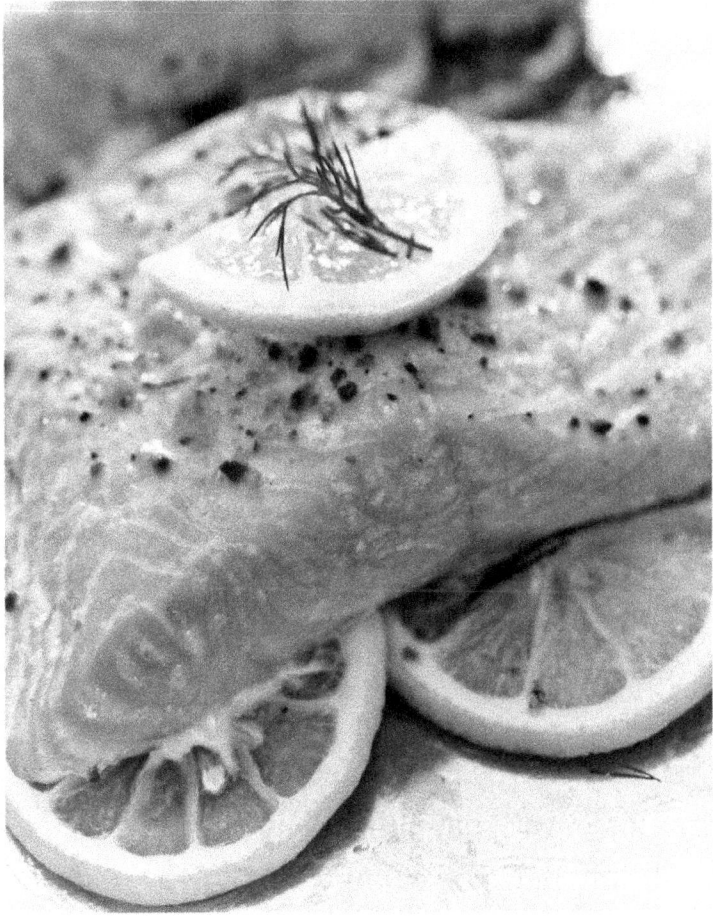

Baked Walnut & Lemon Crusted Salmon

Yield: 4 servings
Preparation Time: 15 minutes
Cooking Time: twenty minutes

Ingredients:

- 1 cup walnuts
- 1 tablespoon fresh dill, chopped
- 2 tablespoons fresh lemon rind, grated
- ½ teaspoon garlic salt
- Freshly ground black pepper, to taste
- 1 tbsp olive oil
- 3-4 tablespoons Dijon mustard
- 4 (3-ounce) salmon fillets
- 4 teaspoons fresh lemon juice

Directions:

1. Preheat the oven to 350 degrees F. Line a substantial baking sheet with parchment paper. 2. In a mixer, add walnuts and pulse till chopped roughly.

3. Add dill, lemon rind, garlic salt, black pepper and oil and pulse till a crumbly mixture forms. 4. Place the salmon fillets, skin-side onto the prepared baking sheet in a very single layer.

5. Coat the surface of each salmon fillet with Dijon mustard evenly.

6. Place the walnut mixture over each fillet evenly and gently, press into the surface of salmon.

7. Bake for about 15-20 min.

8. Serve with the drizzling of fresh lemon juice

Baked Cheesy Salmon

Yield: 4 servings

Preparation Time: 15 minutes

Cooking Time: 25 minutes

Ingredients:

- 2 garlic cloves, crushed
- 1 teaspoon dried dill weed, crushed
- Salt and freshly ground black pepper, to taste
- 2 pounds salmon fillets
- 1 cup cheddar cheese, shredded
- 6 scallions, chopped

Directions:

1. Preheat the oven to 450 degrees F.

2. In a bowl, mix together garlic, dill weed, salt and black pepper.

3. Sprinkle the salmon fillets with garlic mixture evenly.

4. Arrange the salmon fillets over a big foil paper and fold to seal.

5. Place the salmon parcel in a very baking sheet and bake approximately twenty minutes.

6. Now, unfold the parcel and top the salmon fillets with cheese and scallions.

7. Bake for about 5 minutes.

Grilled Salmon with Peach & Onion

Yield: 4 servings

Preparation Time: fifteen minutes

Cooking Time: 12 minutes

Ingredients:
- 4 salmon steak
- Salt and freshly ground black pepper, to taste
- 3 peaches, pitted and cut into wedges
- 2 medium red onions, cut into wedges
- 1 tablespoon fresh ginger, minced
- 1 teaspoon fresh thyme leaves, minced
- 3 tablespoons essential olive oil
- 1 tablespoon balsamic vinegar

Directions:
1. Preheat the grill to medium heat. Grease the grill grate.

2. Sprinkle the salmon with salt and black pepper evenly.

3. In a bowl, add peach, onion, salt and black pepper and toss to coat well.

4. Grill the salmon steaks for approximately 5-6 minutes.

5. Now, place peaches and onions on the grill with salmon steaks.

6. Grill the salmon for about 5-6 minutes per side.

7. Grill the peaches and onion for around 3-4 minutes per side.

8. Meanwhile in a bowl, add remaining ingredients and mix till a smooth paste forms.

9. Place ginger mixture over salmon filets evenly and serve with peaches and onions.

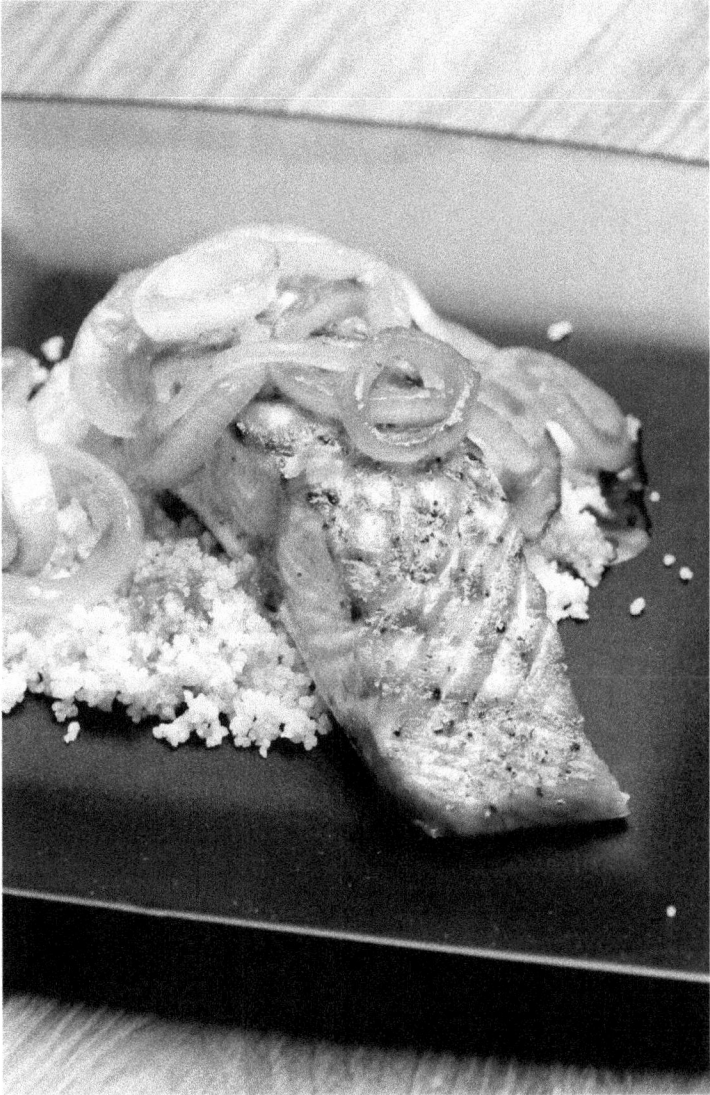

Shrimp Curry Delicious

Yield: 4 servings
Preparation Time: 15 minutes
Cooking Time: 18 minutes

Ingredients:
- 2 tablespoons peanut oil
- ½ sweet onion, minced
- 2 minced garlic cloves
- 1½ teaspoons ground turmeric
- 1 teaspoon ground cumin
- 1 teaspoon ground ginger
- 1 teaspoon paprika
- ½ teaspoon red chili powder
- 1 (14-ounce) can coconut milk
- 1 (14 ½-ounce) can chopped tomatoes
- Salt, to taste
- 1 pound cooked shrimp, peeled and deveined
- 2 tablespoons fresh cilantro, chopped

Directions:
1. In a big skillet, heat oil on medium heat.
2. Add onion and sauté approximately 5 minutes.
3. Reduce the temperature to low.
4. Add garlic and spices and sauté for around 1 minute.

5. Add coconut milk, tomatoes and salt and simmer for about 10 min, stirring occasionally.
6. Stir in the shrimp and cilantro and simmer approximately 1-2 minutes.

Salmon in Spicy Yogurt Gravy

Yield: 5-6 servings
Preparation Time: 15 minutes
Cooking Time: 35 minutes

Ingredients:

- 5-6 salmon steaks
- 1½ teaspoons ground turmeric, divided
- Salt, to taste
- 3 tablespoons coconut oil, divided
- 1 (1-inch) stick cinnamon, pounded roughly
- 3-4 green cardamom, pounded roughly
- 4-5 whole cloves, pounded roughly
- 2 bay leaves
- 1 onion, chopped finely
- 1 teaspoon garlic paste
- 1½ teaspoons ginger paste
- 3-4 green chilies, halved
- 1 teaspoon red chili powder
- ¾ cup plain Greek yogurt
- ¾ cup water
- Chopped fresh cilantro, for garnishing

Directions:

1. In a bowl, season the salmon with ½ teaspoon of the turmeric and salt and make aside.

2. In a big skillet, melt 1coconut oil on medium heat.

3. Add salmon and cook approximately 2-3 minutes per side.

4. Transfer the salmon right into a bowl.

5. In the identical skillet, melt remaining oil on medium heat.

6. Add cinnamon, green cardamom, whole cloves and bay leaves and sauté for around 1 minute.

7. Add onion and sauté for about 4-5 minutes.

8. Add garlic paste, ginger paste, green chilies and sauté for about 2 minutes.

9. Reduce the warmth to medium-low.

10. Add remaining turmeric, red chili powder and salt and sauté for about 1 minute.

11. Meanwhile in a very bowl, add yogurt and water and beat till smooth.

12. Now, slow up the heat to low and slowly, add the yogurt mixture, stirring continuously.

13. Simmer, covered for about fifteen minutes.

14. Carefully, add the salmon fillets and simmer for approximately 5 minutes.

15. Serve hot using the topping of cilantro.

Mango Salad

Yield: 6 servings

Preparation Time: fifteen minutes

Ingredients:
For Dressing:
- 1 fresh Serrano chile, chopped
- 1 tablespoon fresh cilantro, chopped
- 1 teaspoon fresh ginger, chopped
- ¼ cup golden raisins, soaked in boiling water approximately half an hour and drained
- 3 tablespoons extra virgin organic olive oil
- 2 tablespoons balsamic vinegar
- Salt, to taste

For Salad:
- 8 cups fresh mixed baby greens
- 1 medium red bell pepper, seeded and sliced thinly
- 1 large mango, peeled, pitted and cubed

Directions:
1. For dressing in a very blender, add all ingredients and pulse till smooth.
2. Reserve 1 tablespoon of the dressing.
3. In a large bowl, squeeze greens and remaining dressing and toss to coat well.

4. In another bowl, add bell pepper, mango and reserved dressing and toss to coat.

5. Divide the greens and mango mixture in serving bowls.

6. Serve immediately

Lemony Fruit Salad

Yield: 16 servings
Preparation Time: 25 minutes

Ingredients:
- 1 fresh pineapple, peeled, cored and chopped
- 2 large mangoes, peeled, pitted and chopped
- 2 large Fuji apples, cored and chopped
- 2 large red Bartlett pears, cored and chopped
- 2 large navel oranges, peeled, seeded and sectioned
- 2 teaspoons fresh ginger, grated finely
- 2 tablespoons organic honey
- ¼ cup fresh lemon juice

Directions:
1. In a big bowl, mix together all fruits.

2. In a little bowl, add remaining ingredients and beat well.

3. Place honey mixture over fruit mixture and toss to coat well.

4. Refrigerate, covered till chilled completely.

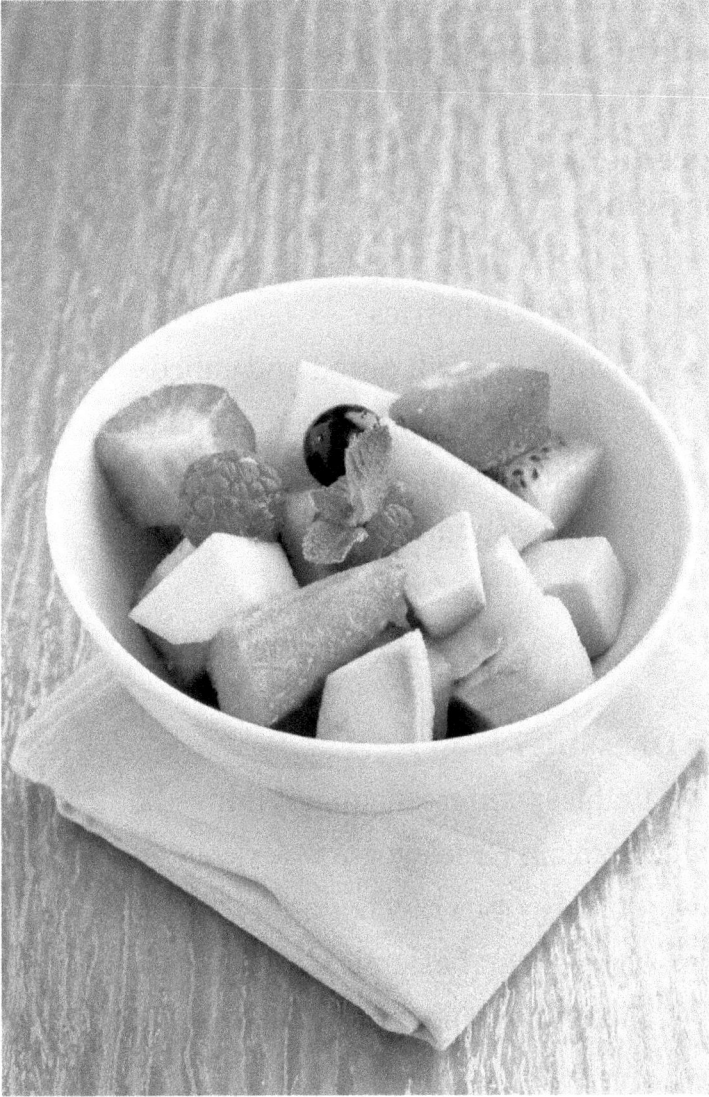

Wheat Berries & Mango Salad

Yield: 4 servings

Preparation Time: 20 minutes

Cooking Time: 35 minutes

Ingredients:

For Salad:

- 2 cups water
- 1 cup wheat berries
- 1 mango, peeled, pitted and cubed
- ½ of red bell pepper, seeded and chopped
- 2 scallions, chopped
- ½ cup fresh mint leaves, chopped
- ½ cup cranberries
- ½ cup walnuts, toasted and chopped

For Dressing:

- 1 tablespoon fresh ginger, minced
- cup plain Greek yogurt
- 3 tablespoons raw honey
- ½ teaspoon balsamic vinegar
- Salt and freshly ground black pepper, to taste

Directions:

1. In a pan, add water and warmth berries and bring to your boil.

2. Cover and cook for approximately 35 minutes.

3. Remove from heat whilst aside for cooling.

4. In a large bowl, add wheat berries and remaining ingredients and mix.

5. In a little bowl, add dressing ingredients and beat well.

6. Place dressing over fruit mixture and toss to coat well.

7. Serve immediately.

Berries & Watermelon Salad

Yield: 8-10 servings

Preparation Time: 20 min

Ingredients:

- 2½ pound seedless watermelon, cubed
- 2 cartons fresh strawberries, hulled and sliced
- 2 cups fresh blueberries
- 1 tablespoon fresh ginger root, grated
- ¼- ounce fresh mint leaves, chopped
- 1 tablespoon raw honey
- ¼ cup fresh lime juice

Directions:

1. In a sizable bowl, mix together all ingredients.
2. Serve immediately.

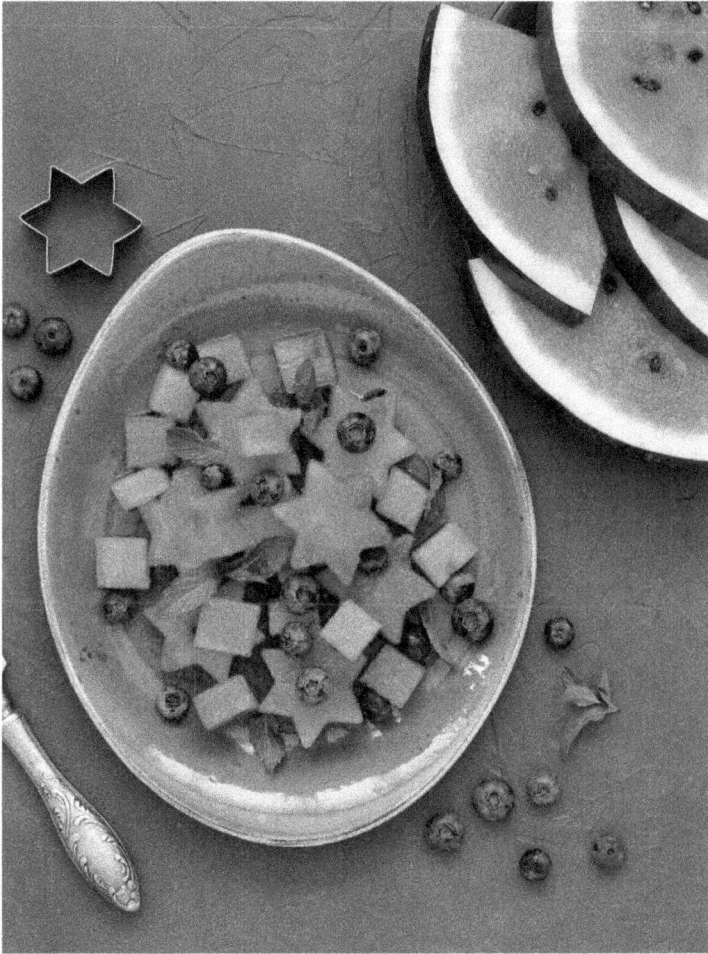

Pear & Jicama Salad

Yield: 4 servings

Preparation Time: quarter-hour

Ingredients:
For Salad:

- 2 small pears, cored and sliced thinly
- 1 pound jicama, sliced into matchsticks
- 1 sprig fresh mint
- 1 sprig fresh parsley

For Dressing:

- 2 tablespoons extra virgin olive oil
- 3 tablespoons fresh orange juice
- 1 tablespoon using apple cider vinegar
- ¼ teaspoon ginger powder
- Salt, to taste

Directions:

1. In a big bowl, mix together all salad ingredients.
2. In a smaller bowl, add dressing ingredients and beat well.
3. Place dressing over salad mixture and toss to coat well.
4. Serve immediately.

Carrot & Almond Salad

Yield: 4 servings

Preparation Time: 15 minutes

Ingredients:

- 1 garlic clove, minced
- 2 teaspoons fresh ginger, grated finely
- ¼ cup coconut milk
- 2 tablespoons almond butter
- 2 tablespoons coconut aminos
- 1 tablespoon fresh lemon juice
- Pinch of cayenne
- Salt, to taste
- 5 large carrots, peeled and grated
- Chopped almonds, to taste

Directions:

1. In a large bowl, add all ingredients except carrots and almonds and mix till well combined. 2. Add carrots and stir to mix.

3. Serve with the garnishing of almonds.

Beet, Carrot & Parsley Salad

Yield: 5 servings

Preparation Time: 15 minutes

Ingredients:
For Salad:
- 1 cup Daikon radishes, trimmed, peeled and julienned
- 3 cups carrots, peeled and julienned
- ½ cup fresh parsley, chopped

For Dressing:
- 1 teaspoon fresh ginger, grated finely
- 2 tablespoons balsamic vinegar
- 1 tablespoon extra-virgin extra virgin olive oil
- 2 teaspoons coconut aminos
- 2 teaspoons raw honey
- ¼ teaspoon granulated garlic
- Salt, to taste

Directions:
1. In a big bowl, mix together all salad ingredients.
2. In a tiny bowl, add dressing ingredients and beat well.
3. Place dressing over fruit mixture and toss to coat well.
4. Serve immediately.

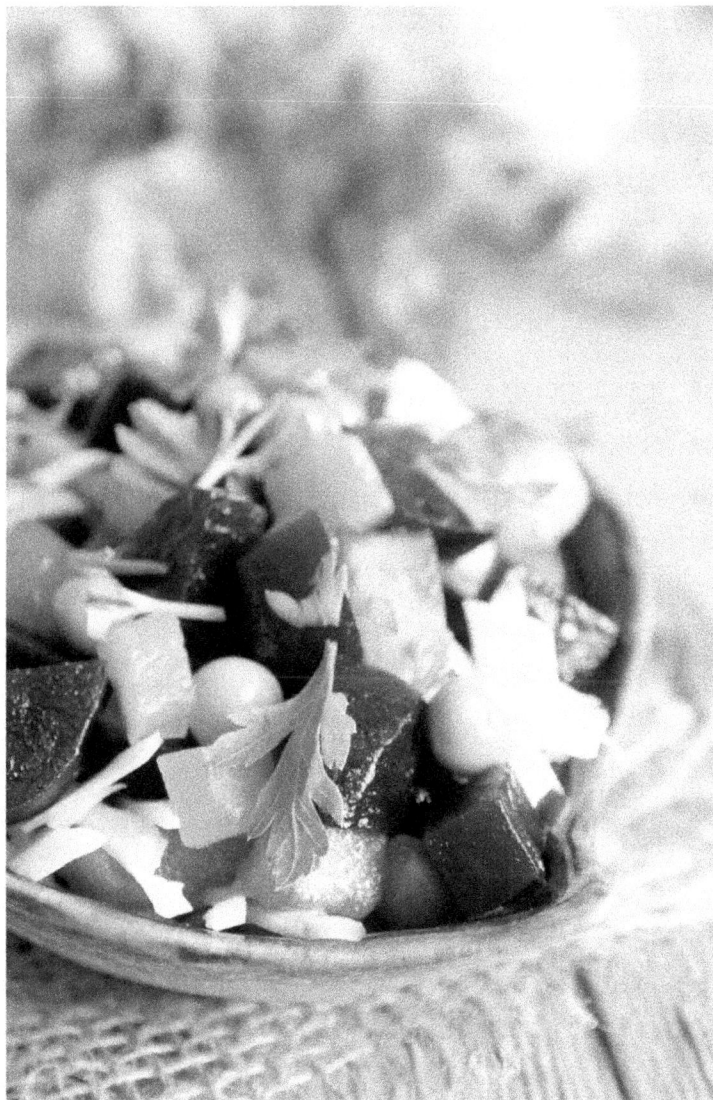

Greens & Seeds Salad

Yield: 4 servings
Preparation Time: 20 minutes
Cooking Time: 6 minutes

Ingredients:
- 1½ teaspoons fresh ginger, grated finely
- 2 tablespoons apple cider vinegar treatment
- 3 tablespoons olive oil
- 1 teaspoon sesame oil, toasted
- 3 teaspoons raw honey, divided
- ½ teaspoon red pepper flakes, crushed and divided
- Salt, to taste
- 1 tablespoon water
- 2 tablespoons raw sunflower seeds
- 1 tablespoon raw sesame seeds
- 1 tablespoon raw pumpkin seeds
- 10-ounce collard greens, stems and ribs removed and thinly sliced leaves

Directions:
1. For dressing inside a bowl, add ginger, vinegar, both oils, 1 teaspoon of honey, ¼ teaspoon red pepper flakes and salt and bat till well combined. Keep aside.
2. In another bowl, add remaining honey, remaining red pepper flakes and water and mix till well combined.
3. Heat a medium nonstick skillet on medium heat.

4. Add all seeds and cook, stirring for approximately 3 minutes.

5. Stir in honey mixture and cook, stirring continuously for about 3 minutes.

6. Transfer the seeds mixture onto parchment paper and set aside to cool down completely.

7. Break the seeds mixture into small pieces.

8. In a large bowl, add the greens, 2 teaspoons with the dressing plus a little salt and toss to coat well.

9. With both your hands, rub the greens for around a few seconds.

10. Add remaining dressing and toss to coat well.

11. Serve with a garnish of seeds pieces.

Cucumber Salad

Yield: 4 servings
Preparation Time: 10 min

Ingredients:
For Salad:

- 2 cucumbers, spiralized with blade C
- 1 avocado, peeled, pitted and sliced
- 2-3 green onions, sliced
- Toasted sesame seeds, as required

For Dressing:

- 1 teaspoon fresh ginger, grated finely
- 1 garlic clove, minced
- 1 teaspoon raw honey
- 1 tablespoon coconut aminos
- 1 tablespoon sesame oil, toasted
- 1 tbsp olive oil

Directions:
1. In a large bowl, squeeze cucumber pasta.
2. In another small bowl, add all dressing ingredients and beat till well combined.
3. Place dressing over cucumber and toss to coat well.
4. Serve with all the topping of remaining ingredients.

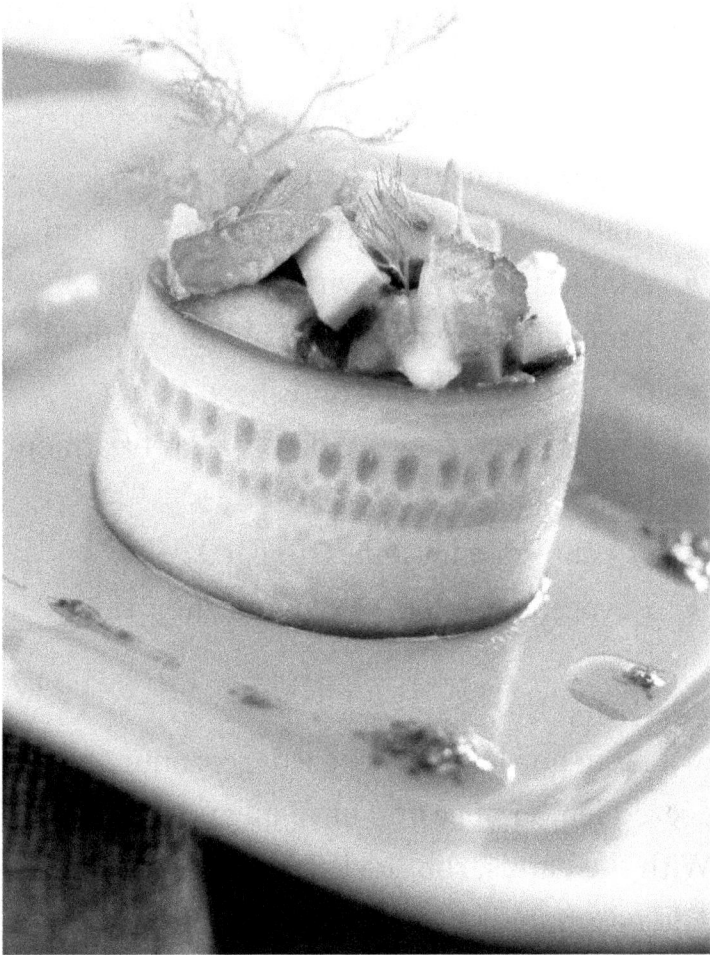

Kale, Carrot & Radish Salad

Yield: 4 servings

Preparation Time: 10 min

Ingredients:

- 1 bunch fresh kale, trimmed and sliced thinly
- 1 large garlic herb, minced
- 2 tablespoons coconut aminos
- 2 tablespoons fresh lemon juice
- 1 tablespoon extra-virgin organic olive oil
- 2 tablespoons extra-virgin coconut oil
- 2 medium carrots, peeled and sliced thinly
- 6 radishes, trimmed and sliced thinly
- 2 tablespoons apple cider vinegar treatment
- Salt, to taste
- 1/3 cup coconut flakes, toasted
- 1 avocado, peeled, pitted and chopped

Directions:

1. In a large bowl, add kale, garlic, coconut aminos, freshly squeezed lemon juice and olive oil and toss to coat well.

2. With the hands, rub the kale generously.

3. Add coconut oil and toss to coat well.

4. Keep aside for about quarter-hour, stringing occasionally.

5. In another bowl, mix together the carrots, radishes and vinegar and keep aside for around quarter-hour, stirring occasionally.

6. Add the carrot mixture inside the bowl with kale mixture and toss to combine.

7. Serve using a garnishing of coconut flakes and avocado.

Citrus Mixed Veggie Salad

Yield: 4 servings

Preparation Time: 20 minutes

Ingredients:

For Salad:

- ½ of the cabbage head, sliced thinly
- 2 carrots, peeled and cut into matchsticks
- 1 zucchini, peeled and cut into matchsticks
- 1 raw beetroot, peeled and cut into matchsticks
- 1 red bell pepper, seeded and sliced thinly
- 2 scallions, sliced thinly
- 3 tablespoons cashews, toasted
- 2 tablespoons sunflower seeds, toasted
- Lime wedges, for serving

For Dressing:

- 3 tablespoons cashews, toasted
- 2 tablespoons sunflower seeds, toasted
- 1 large thumb size piece fresh ginger, chopped
- ½ cup fresh cilantro
- ¼ cup fresh mint leaves
- 2 tablespoons fresh lime juice •
- 2 tablespoons fresh lemon juice
- 1 tbsp essential olive oil

Directions:
1. In a big bowl, mix together all salad ingredients except cashews, sunflower seeds and lime wedges.
2. In a smaller bowl, add dressing ingredients and beat well.
3. Place dressing over salad mixture and toss to coat well.
4. Serve immediately with the garnishing of cashews, sunflower seeds alongside the lime wedges.

Warm Chickpeas Salad

Yield: 4 servings
Preparation Time: 10 min
Cooking Time: 10 min

Ingredients:
- 5 tablespoons virgin olive oil
- 1 large red onion, chopped finely
- 2 minced garlic cloves
- 2 (15-ounce) cans chickpeas, rinsed and drained
- Pinch of red pepper flakes, crushed
- ½ teaspoon ground ginger
- 1 tablespoon freshly squeezed lemon juice
- Salt and freshly ground black pepper, to taste
- ¼ teaspoon paprika
- ½ teaspoon ground cumin
- 2 tablespoons fresh cilantro, chopped

Directions:
1. In a skillet, heat 1 tablespoon of oil on medium-low heat.
2. Add onion and garlic and sauté for approximately 5-7 minutes.
3. Add chickpeas, red pepper flakes and ground ginger and cook approximately 1 minute.
4. Add fresh lemon juice and cook for around 1-2 minutes or till each of the liquid is absorbed.
5. Transfer the chickpea mixture in the serving bowl.

6. Add remaining oil, paprika and cumin and gently, stir to blend.

7. Serve warm using the garnishing of cilantro.

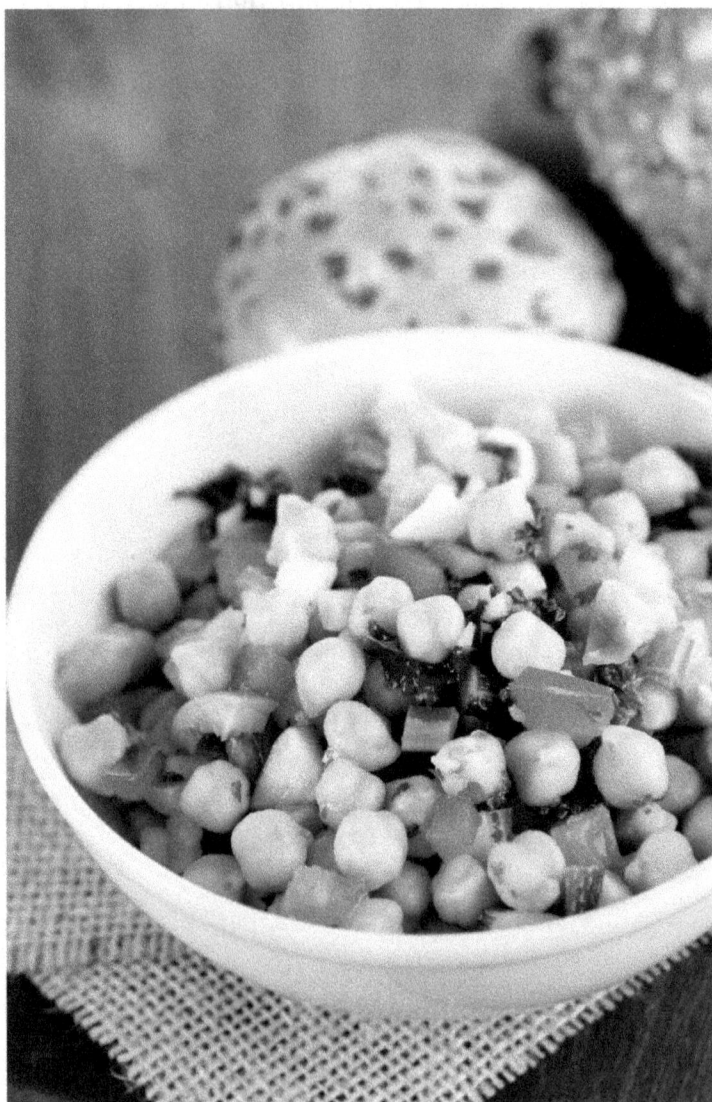

Black Beans & Mango Salad

Yield: 6 servings
Preparation Time: 15 minutes

Ingredients:
For salad:

- 2 (15½-ounce) cans black beans, rinsed and drained
- 2 mangoes, peeled, pitted and chopped
- ½ cup red onion, chopped
- 2 tablespoons fresh cilantro, chopped

For Dressing:

- 1 (½-inch) pieces fresh ginger, grated
- 2 teaspoons fresh orange zest, grated finely
- 3-4 tablespoons fresh orange juice
- 1 tablespoon using apple cider vinegar
- 2 teaspoons extra-virgin olive oil
- ¼ teaspoon red pepper flakes, crushed

Directions:

1. In a large bowl, mix together all salad ingredients.
2. In another bowl, add all dressing ingredients and beat till well combined.
3. Place dressing over beans mixture and mix till well combined.
4. Serve immediately.

Lentil & Beet Salad

Yield: 2-3 servings

Preparation Time: quarter-hour

Cooking Time: twenty or so minutes

Ingredients:
For Salad:

- 2¾ cups water
- 1 cup puy lentils, rinsed
- Salt, to taste
- 3 cooked beetroots, peeled and cubed
- 2 scallions, chopped
- 2 tablespoons fresh parsley, chopped
- 2 tablespoons fresh mint leaves, chopped
- 2 tablespoons hazelnuts, chopped

For Dressing:

- 1 (¾-inch) piece fresh ginger, chopped
- 1 teaspoon Dijon mustard
- 1/3 cup extra-virgin essential olive oil
- 1 tablespoon using apple cider vinegar
- Salt and freshly ground black pepper, to taste

Directions:

1. In a sizable pan, add water, lentils and salt on high heat and bring with a boil.

2. Reduce the heat to low and simmer for about 15-twenty minutes or till each of the liquid is absorbed.

3. Transfer the lentils right into a large bowl and set aside to cool down completely.

4. Add remaining salad ingredients and mix.

5. In another bowl, add all dressing ingredients and beat till well combined.

6. Place dressing over lentils mixture and mix till well combined.

7. Serve immediately.

Nutty Chicken Salad

Yield: 6-8 servings

Preparation Time: twenty minutes

Ingredients:
For dressing:
- 2-3 tablespoons plain Greek yogurt
- 3 tablespoons Dijon mustard
- 2 tablespoons sunflower seeds
- 1 teaspoon kelp powder
- ½-1 teaspoon ground turmeric
- ¼ teaspoon garlic powder
- ¼ teaspoon onion powder
- Salt and freshly ground black pepper, to taste

For Salad:
- 4 cooked chicken breasts, shredded
- 2-3 celery stalks, chopped
- 7-10 sprigs fresh parsley
- 2 tablespoons dried cherries
- 2 tablespoons pecan
- 2 tablespoons slivered almonds

Directions:
1. For dressing inside a bowl, add all dressing ingredients and mix till well combined.

2. In another large bowl, mix together salad ingredients.

3. Pour dressing over salad and toss to coat well.

4. Serve immediately.

Chicken, Bok Choy & Jicama Salad

Yield: 4 servings

Preparation Time: twenty or so minutes

Ingredients:

For Dressing:

- 1 tablespoon fresh ginger, chopped
- 2 tablespoons coconut cream
- 2 tablespoons fresh lime juice
- 1 tablespoon sesame oil
- 1 tablespoon coconut aminos
- 1 tablespoon fish sauce
- 1 teaspoon stevia powder

For Salad:

- 2 cups grilled chicken, chopped
- 6 baby bok choy, grilled and chopped
- 2 scallions, chopped
- ½ cup jicama, chopped
- ¼ cup fresh cilantro, chopped
- 1 tablespoon sesame seeds

Directions:

1. For dressing in the blender, add all dressing ingredients and mix till well combined.

2. In another large bowl, mix together salad ingredients.

3. Pour dressing over salad and toss to coat well.

4. Serve immediately

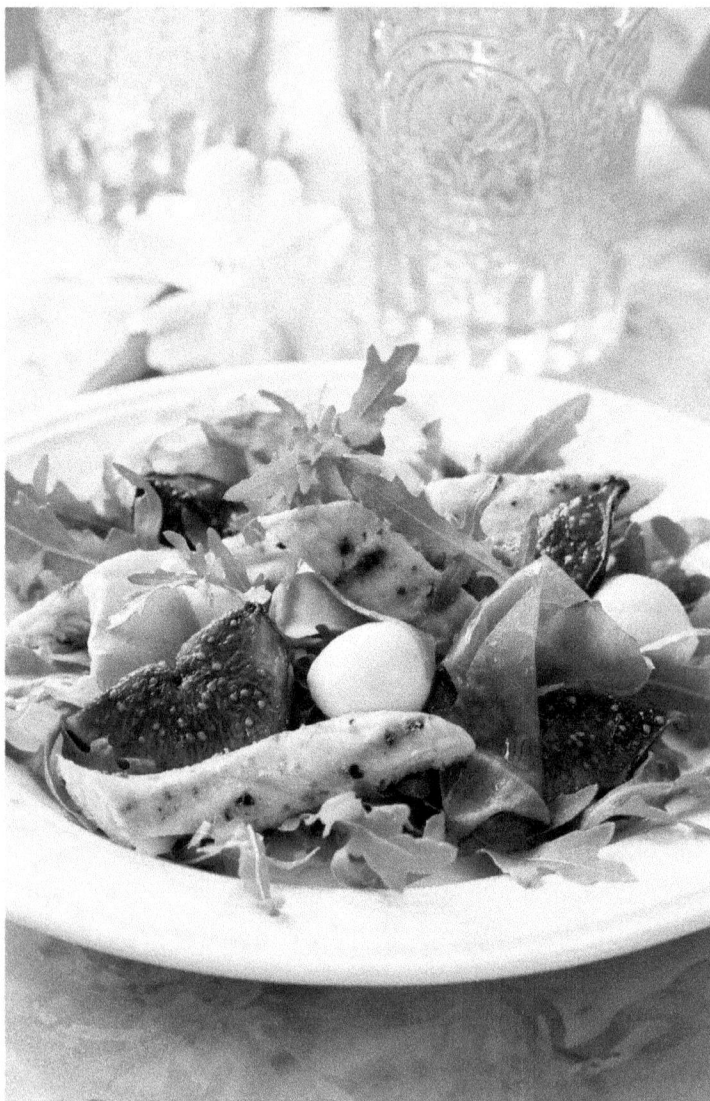

Chicken & Broccolini Salad

Yield: 2 servings
Preparation Time: 25 minutes
Cooking Time: 12 minutes

Ingredients:
For Chicken:
- 1 tablespoon coconut oil
- ½ medium onion, chopped
- 9-ounce boneless chicken thigh, chopped finely
- 1 large garlic herb, minced
- 1 teaspoon fresh lime zest, grated finely
- 1 teaspoon ground turmeric
- 1 teaspoon fresh lime juice
- Salt and freshly ground black pepper, to taste

For Salad:
- 6 broccolini stalks
- 3 large kale leaves, trimmed and chopped
- ½ of avocado, peeled, pitted and chopped
- 2 tablespoons fresh parsley leaves, chopped
- 2 tablespoons fresh cilantro, chopped
- 2 tablespoons pumpkin seeds, toasted

For Dressing:
- 1 small garlic cloves, grated finely

- ½ teaspoon Dijon mustard
- 3 tablespoons extra-virgin olive oil
- 3 tablespoons fresh lime juice
- 1 teaspoon raw honey
- Salt and freshly ground black pepper, to taste

Directions:

1. In a small skillet, melt coconut oil on medium-high heat.

2. Add onion and sauté for approximately 4-5 minutes.

3. Add chicken and garlic and stir fry for about 2-3 minutes.

4. Add remaining ingredients and cook, stirring occasionally approximately 3-4 minutes.

5. Meanwhile in the pan of boiling water, add broccolini and cook for around 2 minutes.

6. Drain well and rinse under cold water and after that cut each stalk in 3-4 pieces.

7. In a bowl, add all dressing ingredients and mix till well combined.

8. Add kale and along with your hands rub till coated with dressing generously.

9. Add chicken, broccolini, avocado, herbs and pumpkin seeds and toss to coat well.

10. Serve immediately.

Notes

www.ingramcontent.com/pod-product-compliance
Lightning Source LLC
Chambersburg PA
CBHW050759030426
42336CB00012B/1875